Reverse and Prevent Heart Disease

Natural Ways to Stop and Prevent Heart Disease, Using Plant-Based, Oil-Free Diets (Cure Congestive Heart Failure)

By

Kim Hilton

Reverse and Prevent Heart Disease

First edition. July, 2018.

Copyright © 2018 Kim Hilton

Written by Kim Hilton

Books by The Same Author

- Boost Your Energy Levels: 60 Natural Ways to Get Rid of Fatigue, Dizziness, Weakness, And Lack of Motivation

- How to Get Rid Of Stretch Marks Naturally

- How to Break Sugar Cravings with Nutritional Supplements: Healthy and Natural Alternatives

- The Anti-Anxiety Cookbook: Nutritional Plan to Cure Depression and Anxiety (Stress Relief and Mental Health Cookpot)

- Eating Disorder Recovery Workbook: How to Recover from

- <u>Natural Treatments for Yeast Infection: How to Cure a Yeast Infection Using Home Remedies</u>
- <u>Itchy Skin Solution: Effective Home Remedies to Get Rid of Dry, Itchy Skin</u>
- <u>Top 30 Cancer-Fighting Foods: Diets and Nutritional Meal Plans to Manage, Overcome, and Prevent Cancer</u>
- <u>Home Remedies for Toothache: Natural Ways to Relieve Severe Toothache and Gum Pain</u>

Table of Contents

Introduction

Your heart tops the list of one of your most hardworking organs in your body and it is also one of your most important organs. It is responsible for pumping oxygenated blood all through your body and it also collects de-oxygenated blood, purifies it and sends it back.

It does this daily, from the time you were born till when you will die. Diseases and impairment in the structures and functions of the heart is life-threatening and can even lead to death when not diagnosed early and treated promptly.

Heart disease is one of the biggest killer diseases on the planet. The term "heart disease" is often used interchangeably with "cardiovascular disease". Cardiovascular disease affects the heart and the blood vessels, while heart disease has to do with the heart only and there are many types of heart disease.

Health complications that can arise from heart disease are heart failure, sudden cardiac arrest, heart attack, peripheral artery disease, stroke and aneurysm, a

condition that leads to internal bleeding.

Causes of Heart Disease

There are various factors that cause heart disease and they are also called the risk factors for this killer disease. The root cause of heart disease is atherosclerosis.

Atherosclerosis is a medical condition characterized by a narrowed or blocked blood vessels. This is mainly caused by buildup of plaques in the blood vessels, as the plaque builds up, the blood vessels become hardened and narrow thereby obstructing the flow of blood to the heart or other parts of the body.

Unhealthy diet, smoking, excessive body weight (obesity), and sedentary lifestyles are risk factors for atherosclerosis. We will take a look at some causes of the different types of heart disease.

Causes of Valvular heart disease are:

- Infections

- Fever (rheumatic fever)

- Disorders of the connective tissues

Causes of abnormal heart beats are:

- Congenital heart disorder

- Heart disease of the valves

- Coronary artery disease

- Some medications and dietary supplements

- Blocked arteries and coronary artery disease

- Stress

- Hypertension

- Abuse and indiscriminate use of legal and illegal drugs

- Diabetes

- Excessive drinking and intake of caffeine

- Smoking

- Electric shock

Causes of infections that lead to heart diseases are pathogens like bacteria, viruses and other parasites can cause endocarditis and other infections the heart. Irritants like chemicals can also lead to infections of the heart.

Causes of congenital heart failure and defects are mainly genetic, it occurs and develops when the baby is still in the womb, it develops when the heart is developing and this is usually one month after conception.

This condition changes the way blood flows in the heart. Factors that play a role in this are genes, vaccines and medications. Congenital heart defect can also happen to adults because as an individual age, the structure of his/her can also change.

Causes of weak heart muscles also known as cardiomyopathy are hereditary, certain medications, toxins, chemicals, diseases, aging and cancer treatments can

cause it.

Risk Factors for Heart Disease

Common risk factors that can lead to the development of heart disease are:

- Unhealthy lifestyles

- Smoking

- Unhealthy diets

- Aging

- Stress

- Sedentary lifestyle and physical inactivity

- Family history and genetics

- Sex

- Some medications, cancer drugs and radiation therapies

- High levels of cholesterol in the bloodstream

- High blood pressure

- Obesity

- Diabetes

- Poor hygiene (raises the risk of infection).

Types of Heart Disease

Cardiomyopathy

Also known as weak heart muscles, there are three types of cardiomyopathy and they are:

1. Restrictive cardiomyopathy:

This type is usually rare and it is characterized by a rigid and less elastic heart muscles. Cancer treatments, excess buildup of proteins (amyloidosis) and iron (hemochromatosis) in the body, and diseases like connective tissue disorder are risk factors for this class of cardiomyopathy.

2. Hypertrophic cardiomyopathy

This type is known by an abnormal thickness of the heart muscles, especially the walls of the left ventricles. It is mostly inherited but aging and high blood pressure can cause this in rare cases and it leads to sudden death.

3. Dilated cardiomyopathy

This is the most common form of cardiomyopathy but the cause is not fully known but it is believed to be caused by coronary artery disease which causes a low supply of oxygen to the muscles of the heart.

It leads to an enlarged left ventricle and the chambers of the heart are dilated due to weak muscles.

It can be inherited; certain drugs, toxins, infections, and ischemic heart disease (reduced flow of blood to the heart) can cause this.

Heart Attack

"A significant part of the muscles of the heart is being impaired when there is shortage of blood supply to the heart. This interruption of the natural flow of blood to the hear leads to heart attack." Blood clot or blood clots in one of the coronary arteries are common causes of heart attack.

This can also be caused by sudden spasms or narrowing of the arteries. This is also called coronary thrombosis or cardiac infarction.

Valvular Heart Disease

This type is characterized by damaged valves, the heart has 4 valves; they are the aortic valve, the tricuspid valve, the pulmonary valve, and the mitral valve.

This condition leads to improper closing of the valves, narrowing of the valves, known as stenosis, or leaking (regurgitations) of the valves. The three main types under this class of heart disease are:

1. Pulmonary stenosis: The heart has difficulty in pumping blood from the right ventricle into the pulmonary artery

due to the tightness of the pulmonary valve.

This makes the right ventricle work harder in order to overcome this obstruction. It does not give symptoms in older kids but infants can turn blue. An open-heart surgery is mostly carried out on the patient to remove this obstruction.

2. Mitral regurgitation: This is caused by the inability of the mitral valve to close tightly; this lets blood flow back into the heart instead of going out.

This affects the circulation of blood in the body and it causes extreme tiredness and breathlessness in those that have this condition.

3. Mitral valve prolapse: This type is not threatening and it does not need treatment.

In this case, the valve that is between the left ventricle and the left atrium does not close fully and it protrudes upwards or backwards into the atrium.

Atherosclerosis Disease of the Heart

This type of heart disease is caused by a blocked blood vessel.

Congenital Heart Disease

This type is genetic and it is evident after birth, adults can also develop this and this is caused by aging. There are various forms of congenital heart defects and some of them are:

1. Cyanotic heart disease which reduces the levels of oxygen in the body.

2. Septal defects are characterized by a hole inbetween the chambers of your heart.

3. Obstruction defects are characterized by an obstruction or a total blockage of the blood flow through the chambers of the heart.

Heart Arrhythmias

This heart disease is characterized by irregular and abnormal heartbeat. This occurs when the electric impulses do not function properly, these electrical impulses help to coordinate the heartbeats.

There are various types of arrhythmia and this is classified based on the way your heart beats. Fibrillation is defined by irregular heartbeat, tachycardia is defined as rapid heartbeat and Bradycardia is defined by a low heartbeat.

Premature ventricular contractions also cause abnormal heartbeats. Heart arrhythmias can be fatal.

Heart Disease Caused by Infections

Parasites and pathogens like bacteria, and viruses can cause this type of heart disease. An example of this is endocarditis, this is an infection of the heart that impairs the inner membrane separating the chambers of the heart.

Coronary Artery Disease

Your heart and its muscles are given nutrients and oxygenated blood via the coronary arteries. When these arteries are diseased or damaged, this leads to less supply of oxygenated blood and nutrients to the heart.

Plaque deposits inside your coronary arteries can cause this.

Congestive Heart Failure

Also known as heart failure, it occurs when the heart experiences difficulties in pumping blood all through the body. Either sides of the heart can be affected but it is not common for the two sides of the heart to be affected.

This can be induced by high blood pressure or coronary artery disease, these conditions make the heart very weak or too stiff to accumulate and pump blood

effectively.

Symptoms of Heart Disease

These symptoms are based on the type and they are different for both sexes.

For instance, in atherosclerosis, (heart disease of the blood vessels), men experience only chest pain while women experience other signs and discomforts besides chest pain and some of them are shortness of breath, extreme tiredness and weaknesses, discomforts in the chest and nausea.

Other symptoms of atherosclerosis include:

•	Pains in some parts of the body like the back, upper abdomen, neck, throat or jaw.

•	Tightness in the chest, and angina (chest pain, chest pressure and chest discomfort).

•	Shortness of breath

•	Pain, weaknesses and numbness in some parts of the body,

- Cold hands and feet signifying blocked or narrowed blood vessels.

Symptoms of heart attack are:

- Heartburn

- Indigestion

- Feeling heavy in your chest

- Stomach ache

- Profuse sweating

- Pains all over your body

- Dizziness, nausea and vomiting

Symptoms of Valvular heart disease (diseases that affects the four valves of the heart) depend on the affected or damaged valve. But the general symptoms include:

- Regular episodes of fainting

- Extreme fatigue and tiredness

- Chest pain

- Shortness of breath

- Swollen ankles and feet

- Irregular heartbeat

Symptoms of heart arrhythmias (abnormal heartbeats) are:

- Fainting or near fainting

- Fluttering inside your chest

- Dizziness

- Fast heartbeat also known as tachycardia

- Lightheadedness

- Slow heartbeat also known as Bradycardia

- Shortness of breath

- Chest discomforts and chest pain

Symptoms of heart disease caused by infections are:

- Abnormal spots and rashes

- High body temperature and fever

- A dry and persistent cough

- Shortness of breath

- Abnormal heart beat or changes in the rhythm of your heart

- Fatigue and weaknesses

- Swellings in your abdomen and also in your legs

Symptoms of congenital heart disease (this is a term used to refer to heart disease or defects from birth) are:

- Infants experience weight loss, and shortness of breath when they are eating

- Clubbed fingernails

- Extreme fatigue

- Cyanosis and pale complexion like blue skin and pale grey complexion.

- Sweating and rapid heartbeat

•   Swelling of the areas around the eyes, and swelling of the abdomen and legs.

•   Rapid breathing and chest pain

•   Getting tired very easily after a little exercise or activity

•   Difficulty breathing during a physical activity or exercise

Symptoms of heart disease caused by dilated cardiomyopathy (that is a term for weak heart muscles) are:

•   Fainting and lightheadedness

- Dizziness

- Breathlessness that happens at rest and with exertion

- Irregular heartbeat that can be fast, fluttering or pounding

- Swellings of the feet, legs and ankles

- Extreme fatigue and tiredness.

Prevention of Heart Disease

It is not possible to prevent congenital heart disease but other forms of cardiovascular disease are preventable. Make healthy living your lifestyle and you will prevent heart disease from occurring. Healthy lifestyles to imbibe are:

- Quit smoking and avoid tobacco smoke

- Practice good hygiene

• Control your blood pressure, and the levels of glucose and cholesterol in your body.

• Reduce stress or manage it effectively

• Your meals should be low in salt (sodium chloride) and saturated fats

• Exercise daily and engage in lots of physical activities

• Maintain a healthy weight.

- Eat healthy foods always. Include plenty fruits, vegetables and herbs in your daily meals.

How to Reverse Heart Disease

Live a healthy lifestyle

This includes regular intake of healthy meals and dropping bad habits like smoking, excessive drinking and use of illegal drugs or abuse of prescription drugs.

Even if you are genetically predisposed to this disease, these lifestyle changes will help prevent it from happening. Unhealthy foods like junks, processed foods and unnatural foods trigger inflammations in the body and this is a risk factor for heart disease.

Foods that trigger inflammation should be avoided and cut out of your meals, some of them are: Trans fats and hydrogenated oils, corn and soybean oils, all kinds of sugar and artificial sweeteners, conventional and pasteurized diary, conventional meats, processed or refined carbohydrates and many others.

Your meals should be made of whole foods, lots of fruits, herbs, vegetables and plenty water. This will prevent heart disease and improve your general health. Their dense content of antioxidants and phytochemicals fights inflammation and they also boost the immune system.

Citrus Fruits and Juices

Every morning, take citrus fruits and juices like lemons, oranges, grapefruits and others; this will improve the health of your heart and your whole body at large.

Oranges and orange juice cut the risk of heart disease by reducing the levels of homocysteine, this amino acid can trigger a heart attack.

Grapefruit and its juice are rich in resveratrol and flavonoids; these compounds prevent the clumping together of red blood cells and stops the formation of blood clots that can block a blood vessel and lead to heart disease or stroke.

Don't add sugar to their juices.

Hibiscus

Hibiscus flowers fight atherosclerosis. They also contain powerful antioxidants that expel bad cholesterol from the body that leads to heart disease and atherosclerosis.

You can take unsweetened drink daily because sugar can trigger inflammation and make this treatment less effective.

Garlic

This cuts down the risk of heart disease by reducing blood pressure, the levels of cholesterol and even preventing heart disease from occurring when taken regularly.

It prevents the development of atherosclerosis by inhibiting the buildup of plaques in the arteries, thereby preventing hardening or obstruction of the arteries.

It also boosts blood circulation all through the body and it prevents the formation of blood clots which can block a blood vessel and cause heart disease and other complications like stroke.

Eat at least four cloves of garlic daily but those on blood thinning medications should avoid garlic.

Turmeric

Regular consumption of turmeric keeps atherosclerosis at bay. Its active chemical, Curcumin, brings down the levels of cholesterol, it prevents the formation of blood clots and the buildup of plaques in the blood vessels.

It also decreases the levels of bad cholesterol and it fights inflammations. It fights free radicals which are behind aging and lots of chronic diseases like heart disease.

You can take a cup of turmeric tea three times daily. Curcumin supplements are available in health stores, you can get it and take it according to the stipulated dosage.

Exercise Regularly

Regular exercise and increased rate of physical activity prevents the effects of a sedentary lifestyle. It improves the flow of blood to the heart and other parts of the body, it prevents hormonal problems, it supplies more oxygen to your cells and it controls the levels of sugar in your bloodstream and it also helps you feel good and relax.

It is also a good way to prevent your arteries from getting clogged.

Capsaicin

Impairments related to the circulatory system and the heart is also treated using cayenne pepper. "This ingredient is the most active and it is referred to as the Capsaicin." It prevents and reduces the risks of irregular heartbeat and it brings down high levels of cholesterol in your bloodstream.

It also purifies your blood and boosts your immune system, thereby, cutting the risks for infections of the heart. Add a teaspoon of cayenne pepper to a glass of warm water and drink after stirring it very well.

Do this three times daily. Cayenne supplements, capsules, and tablets are also available.

Hawthorn

Due to its excellent effect on the heart, this herb is well known for treating lots of heart problems and it is great for the cardiovascular system.

It increases the flow of blood to the heart and strengthens weak muscles of the heart and helps its contractions thereby leading to optimum pumping and functions of the heart.

It reduces the work done by the heart by preventing these problems and it helps maintains a normal and regular heartbeat.

It is available in supplements, and you can take it according to the dose.

Fenugreek

This remedy protects the heart because it is dense in antioxidants. It cuts the risk of atherosclerosis and it even regulates the concentration of lipids in the bloodstream.

It stops the aggregation of platelets, thus, reducing the risk of blood clots obstructing the blood vessels which can lead to strokes and heart attacks.

It eliminates excess fats from the body, it reduces the levels of glucose and cholesterol in the body. Drink fenugreek tea daily and you should also take it before eating or drinking anything every morning.

Avoid or Reduce Stress

Stress raises the levels of cortisol in the bloodstream and this, in turn, will trigger inflammation, and when not managed properly, it can lead to heart disease.

Chronic stress is caused by lack of proper sleep and rest, working too hard, and our fast-paced lifestyle. "Ginger is an adaptogenic herb which could be taken in tea in order to relax and get rid of stress."

Also, try and get proper sleep, spend time in nature and you can try meditating or praying and also spend a good time with your family and even pets.

Alfalfa

This herb does wonders for the heart, it prevents the buildup of plaques in the arteries, it reduces the levels of bad cholesterol and prevents many types of cardiovascular disease.

It slows the advancement of atherosclerosis in those that already have it. Drink alfalfa tea three times daily or drink its juice mixed with equal amount of water many times daily, till you see positive results.

The supplements are also available.

Arjuna

This is an important herb used in Ayurveda medicine for heart problems. It strengthens the muscles of the heart and it reduces angina attacks by thirty percent.

It is a natural tonic for the heart, it prevents hardening and congestion of the arteries and it also lowers high blood pressure, thereby, preventing or treating heart disease.

Pour a teaspoon of Arjuna tree bark powder into a cup of hot water, you can add little honey for taste. Drink this three times daily for some months. You can also buy as supplements and capsules.

Green Tea

There are lots of antioxidants in green tea, it improves the health of the heart and brings down high levels of triglycerides and cholesterol.

It boosts your metabolism and helps you control your sugar levels. Stroke and heart diseases can be tactically prevented by the daily intake of green tea. 8-cups is the recommended dose; by which you can always split them though the day. 26% likeliness of stroke and heart attack is being reduced with the daily dosage of green tea.

Take many cups of green tea daily to prevent and reduce the risks of heart disease.

Other Books by The Same Author

- <u>Boost Your Energy Levels: 60 Natural Ways to Get Rid of Fatigue, Dizziness, Weakness, And Lack of Motivation</u>

- <u>How to Get Rid Of Stretch Marks Naturally</u>

- <u>How to Break Sugar Cravings with Nutritional Supplements: Healthy and Natural Alternatives</u>

- <u>The Anti-Anxiety Cookbook: Nutritional Plan to Cure Depression and Anxiety (Stress Relief and Mental Health Cookpot)</u>

- <u>Eating Disorder Recovery Workbook: How to Recover from Eating Disorder On Your Own (Anorexia, Bulimia Nervosa, And Binge Eating)</u>
- <u>100 Health Hacks Nobody Ever Told You: Natural Tips and Tricks for Enhanced and Prudent Well-Being</u>
- <u>How to Lower Blood Pressure Naturally & Quickly: Powerful Tricks to Deal with Hypertension Using Supplements and Other Natural Remedies</u>
- <u>Reverse Type 2 Diabetes: How to Control and Prevent Diabetes Naturally</u>

- <u>Urinary Tract Infection Treatment: Home Remedies for Urinary Tract Infections and Prevention Methods</u>

- <u>Natural Treatments for Yeast Infection: How to Cure a Yeast Infection Using Home Remedies</u>

- <u>Itchy Skin Solution: Effective Home Remedies to Get Rid of Dry, Itchy Skin</u>

- <u>Top 30 Cancer-Fighting Foods: Diets and Nutritional Meal Plans to Manage, Overcome, and Prevent Cancer</u>

- <u>Home Remedies for Toothache: Natural Ways to Relieve Severe Toothache and Gum Pain</u>

www.ingramcontent.com/pod-product-compliance
Lightning Source LLC
Chambersburg PA
CBHW031427250726
48656CB00002B/861